Routledge Revivals

Defective Housing and the Growth of Children

After World War I, housing was one of many pressing issues facing the country with multiple families often crowded in together in inadequate housing. This had a dramatic impact on health with increasing problems such as tuberculosis and malnutrition. Originally published in 1919, this study aimed to identify the ways in which defective housing impacted on health in the family with a particular focus on rickets in children in the East end of London and the developmental issues resulting from it. This title will be of interest to students of Medical History and Health and Social Care.

Defective Housing and the Growth of Children

J. Lawson Dick

RFF PRESS
RESOURCES FOR THE FUTURE

First published in 1919
by George Allen & Unwin Ltd

This edition first published in 2016 by Routledge
2 Park Square, Milton Park, Abingdon, Oxon, OX14 4RN
and by Routledge
711 Third Avenue, New York, NY 10017

Routledge is an imprint of the Taylor & Francis Group, an informa business

Publisher's Note
The publisher has gone to great lengths to ensure the quality of this reprint but points out that some imperfections in the original copies may be apparent.

Disclaimer
The publisher has made every effort to trace copyright holders and welcomes correspondence from those they have been unable to contact.

A Library of Congress record exists under LC control number: 20009360

ISBN 13: 978-1-138-10052-7 (hbk)
ISBN 13: 978-1-315-65737-0 (ebk)
ISBN 13: 978-1-138-10086-2 (pbk)

DEFECTIVE HOUSING

AND THE

GROWTH OF CHILDREN

BY

J. LAWSON DICK, M.D., F.R.C.S.

Administrative Deputy Commissioner of Medical Services,
Ministry of Pensions, County of London

LONDON: GEORGE ALLEN & UNWIN LTD.
RUSKIN HOUSE, 40 MUSEUM STREET, W.C. 1

First published in 1919

CONTENTS

I

INTRODUCTORY

Defective Housing and the Growth of Children

CHAPTER I

INTRODUCTORY

IN the process of reconstruction after the war there are many problems with which the country is faced which demand a speedy solution. The provision of work for all and a living wage for the worker, providing against periods of ill-health and unemployment, and the failing of the powers with old age, are questions which must be squarely faced and dealt with in a liberal and tolerant spirit. Not only must the worker be granted a living wage, but care must be taken that the expense of living does not increase with the rise in wages. Rents and the prices of foodstuffs must be reasonable, so that the increase in the wage is not annulled by the rise in prices for what are the ordinary necessities of life. The working man must be able to enjoy his fair share of the amenities of life, and his hours of work must be so regulated that he has the opportunity for leisure to employ as he will. His house must not be merely a tenement and a roof to his head, but must be a home where he can rear his children in comfort and provide for their proper development, intellectual, moral, and physical. No one with any knowledge of the more crowded areas in our large towns can pretend that this is possible at the present time. It is a matter of common knowledge that, in the case of a large proportion of our population, families of six persons are herded together in one, two, or three rooms. There is no provision for cooking, which has to be carried on in one of the living rooms, and such a thing as a bath is unknown. Privacy is impossible, and the sleeping accommodation is alien to all ideas of health and ordinary decency. There is no proper means of ventilation, and the air-space round the houses is totally inadequate for the preservation of health. The poetry of life does not exist for these dwellers in the rooms of our mean streets, which stretch for mile upon mile without variation in their squalid misery. In the East End of London, every here and there, there are squares where trees are planted. To allow of the trees living the houses are well set back, permitting the entry of sunlight and fresh air necessary for the growth of the trees. Care is taken that the trees are planted at a sufficient distance from one another to prevent overcrowding, which would stunt their growth. But in the dwellings where young life is to be brought up no such care is taken. Street upon street is crowded one upon another in apparently endless succession, to the exclusion of everything that makes for growth and health. We know that these conditions are inimical to health. An excellent criterion of the unhealthiness of the housing conditions is to be found in the incidence of tuberculosis, which increases in prevalence as the house accommodation becomes more limited and objectionable.

These same conditions which give rise to a high mortality in pulmonary tubercle give rise in a still higher degree to defective growth, both bodily and mental, in the child. With these conditions we naturally tend to have deficient feeding as an associated evil. Intemperance and sloth are encouraged, and a vicious circle is created, till the wonder is, not that things are as bad as they are, but that we should have been able to create out of our mixed population the splendid armies which have been capable of the fine deeds and the physical and mental endurance which they have shown lately in the field. Happily the call for such endurance has not been made on any one class of the population, and it will be strange indeed if, after what all have endured in common, an earnest and tolerant spirit does not arise which will search for and find a way out of the present unequal social conditions, which all must realize ought not to exist. Seven or eight years ago the present enquiry was suggested by a short piece of research work into speech defects occurring amongst school children in London.[1] The essential fact that struck one was the delayed physical and mental development of the children as a whole. Well-marked defects along a definite line were noted which pointed to some constitutional abnormality from which nearly all these children suffered in a greater or less degree. Subsequent research showed that rickets was the prevailing defect from which these children suffered, and that slum dwellings and defective housing were the essential factors in producing this defective growth. Deficiency of sunlight and fresh air and the want of the opportunity for proper exercise of the muscles were the factors which operated in practically all these cases. As will be detailed later on, one thousand children were taken from schools in the East End of London and 80 per cent. of these were found to show definite rickety signs lasting throughout the period of school age. Rickets is not a congenital condition. As a rule, except in the case of congenital syphilis, the

[1] "Speech Defects in School Children." *School Hygiene*, November 1913.

infant, whether it is born in the house of the rich or the house of the very poor, is born healthy. Nature is a kindly mother, and spares no effort to give every child a fair chance. The great enemy to healthy conception and birth is syphilis. This condition is congenital, and the results are so disastrous that as a rule it either destroys the conception before birth, or death follows comparatively soon after birth. Syphilis is not commonly found amongst school children; rickets is excessively common. Apart from syphilis, then, the child is as a rule born healthy, but about six months after birth defects are noticed. The question naturally arises as to how far this is the effect of deficient feeding or bad housing, or both. This is a question of the greatest practical importance at the present time, for if lack of proper feeding is the essential cause of the defective growth of the child the solution of the whole problem is comparatively easy. With our experience of rationing the nation, and with the systematic supervision of the whole population which is being rapidly developed from the ante-natal stage and the earliest infancy to the end of school life, it should be a comparatively simple matter to make sure that no child suffers, as many do at present, from the inadequate supply of cow's milk or whatever other food is necessary for its proper development and growth. But our efforts will to a large extent be wasted if we rest content with this. The essential factor interfering with the normal growth of the child is defective housing. Deficiency of food and errors in dieting will aggravate rickets, but no diet, however efficient, will prevent the occurrence of rickets if the child is brought up under slum conditions. In early infancy, as already stated, the two diseases syphilis and rickets are fairly commonly met with. Both are peculiar in that their effects tend to be indefinitely prolonged if the child survive. Both may run on for years, and the system is profoundly affected at its period of most rapid growth. In both a widespread process of rebuilding or reconstruction takes place which leaves stigmata recognizable especially in the skeleton, skull, and teeth. There are, however, essential differences. Congenital syphilis is due to a micro-organism, whereas in rickets no specific organism is known. Syphilis, as already pointed out, produces a profound toxæmia, so that both the ante-natal and the post-natal mortality is very large, and comparatively few survive to adult life. Rickets, on the other hand, is an eminently curable disease, and tends to end in recovery. It is therefore not only found with great frequency in baby centres, but the stigmata of the disease are exceedingly common in school children and usually persist throughout the whole of the child's school life. So commonly are they found, that it may be stated that practically all children living under the slum conditions which prevail in the East End of London have to struggle through a rickety phase of their existence, during which the whole tide of growth is profoundly disturbed and permanent damage is done to the body tissues and skeleton, and also to the sensitive tissues of the central nervous system.

II

THE STIGMATA OF RICKETS

B

CHAPTER II

THE STIGMATA OF RICKETS

THE following statistics are mainly taken from Jewish schools in the districts of Whitechapel and Stepney. Over eight hundred of the one thousand children examined are Jewish. This is of importance in considering the part played by nutrition of the child in the incidence of rickets. Jewish women make excellent mothers, in so far as their children are well fed and clothed. Indeed, the tendency is to over-clothe the child, and it is often difficult to persuade the mother to discard the extra waistcoats and jerseys with which the child is hampered. But the essential point is that these children do not suffer from cold, bleak winters to the same extent as poorly-clad non-Jewish children. The fat nutrition of these children is usually very good, and yet, in spite of excellent nutrition, rickets is exceedingly common.

Early feeding during infancy.—Of these one thousand children:

81·4 per cent. were breast fed.
18·6 „ „ artificially fed.

Almost all bottle-fed children were brought up on cow's milk; comparatively few Jewish mothers seem to use patent foods or condensed milk. Breast-fed children are children who were suckled on the breast for a period of six months or more; if they were not suckled for six months, they are included amongst the children who were not breast fed. Of children nursed on the breast the following is the duration given in percentage results:

2	per cent.	suckled	from	6	to	9	months.
17	„	„	„	9	„	12	„
61	„	„	„	12	„	18	„
20	„	„	„	18	„	24	

That is, 81 per cent. of these mothers gave their children the breast for periods varying from twelve months to two years.

This prolonged lactation is important, but care must be taken not to exaggerate its influence, as from eight to nine months onwards the mother gives additional food from the general table besides the breast milk. But breast milk is the main support of the child for the first eighteen months or two years. On the other hand, at the Hackney Centre for mothers, where the mothers are almost entirely Christian, out of three hundred mothers attending during the year:

57·5 per cent. nursed their babies entirely on the breast,
20·5 per cent. nursed their babies partly on the breast and partly on the bottle,
22 per cent. were bottle fed.

Unfortunately many of these mothers were out working during the day, and so had to give the baby the bottle during the day, reserving the breast feeding for the night. The Jewish mother seldom goes out to work in this way. Amongst the non-Jewish mothers the use of patent foods, especially condensed milk, is common. Yet even in the case of the Christian mothers the figures show that 78 per cent. nurse their children either wholly or partially on the breast. The poorer classes of mothers, Jewish or Christian, do their duty to their babies in the matter of breast feeding. The fault so far does not lie with the mother.

Of the one thousand children examined:

798 were rickety = 80 per cent.
202 were not rickety = 20 per cent.

It must be understood that these 798 children were not necessarily suffering from rickets at the time of the examination; indeed the majority had recovered, but showed signs of having suffered at one time from rickets, and these rickety stigmata persisted through the child's school life. Rickets is essentially a disease of the first two years of life; but its consequences are far-reaching, and the persistence of the recognizable physical signs affords an index to the lasting damage done to delicate tissues, especially those of the nervous system.

It is still taught that, for all practical

purposes, breast feeding excludes rickets. This is a grave error. Of breast-fed children 72·5 per cent. were rickety; whilst of bottle-fed babies 87 per cent. were rickety. A percentage of 14·5 fewer children showed signs of rickets amongst those who were breast fed; but this still left 72·5 per cent. breast fed who showed evident signs.

Nutrition of the rickety children.—The state of nutrition of those eight hundred children who showed evident signs of rickets may be assessed in three groups:

(1) Of *very good* nutrition, of which there were 23 per cent.

(2) Of *good* nutrition, of which there were 57 per cent.

(3) Of *bad* nutrition, of which there were 20 per cent.

In only one-fifth of these children was the nutrition decidedly poor. This result is very good, and would, in the East End of London, be obtained only in a Jewish school. For this reason Jewish children were purposely selected, for here we have a natural experiment at hand, where good nutrition, notably good fat nutrition, is associated with extremely defective housing conditions as regards want of ventilation, overcrowding and disregard for general cleanliness. But it must not be thought that these figures on the incidence of rickets refer only to Jewish schools. Rickets is equally common in non-Jewish schools, and tends to be of a severer type owing to the association of defective feeding with defective housing conditions. The following were the defects found amongst these children :

Beaded ribs and chest deformities.—The chest signs of rickets are the most common and most constant. Beading of the ribs, if slight and if present alone, was not taken as a sign of rickets, unless there were chest deformities or cranial signs to confirm the diagnosis. In the ordinary inspection of school children beading of the ribs will be found in over 80 per cent. if carefully sought. With this beading of the ribs certain chest deformities are frequently associated. Asymmetry of the chest is common, such as a tendency to flattening at the left apex with a compensatory projection to the right side of the lower part of the sternum, where it meets with the lower true ribs. This is usually the result of a slight lateral curvature, which, in the slighter cases, can often be diagnosed more easily from the front than by examination of the spine itself. Which apex is flattened and which shoulder is elevated will vary with the form of lateral curvature present. It is noteworthy that impairment of the resonance at one or other apex with flattening is frequently due in school children to distortion of the chest and not to tubercle. Another of the slighter deformities of the chest is an elevation of the manubrium sterni at the sterno-clavicular joints, so that the whole chest seems as if it were tilted forwards and raised. The everted edge of the margin of the ribs where pushed outwards by the enlarged abdominal organs, and the associated transverse Harrison's sulcus associated with falling in of the ribs above this margin are well known. Not infrequently the whole sternum is pushed forwards, and the ribs tend to sink in at the sides, to produce the various forms of pigeon breast so characteristic of rickets. When all the ribs are soft the whole sternum projects, and the chest is furrowed laterally as high as the second rib. Not infrequently, however, the upper part of the chest is moderately well expanded, and the somewhat keel-shaped protrusion of the sternum is confined to the lower end, and the retraction of the ribs to the infra-mammary region. The beading of the ribs is probably Nature's attempt to buttress up the weak point at the junction of the ribs with the costal cartilages. The constantly varying strains on this part tend to produce an irritative overgrowth, the result of which becomes palpable very early in the child's life, and which is greater on the inner side of the ribs than it is on the outer.

These defects are common in children not at first suspected of rickets.

Antero-posterior flattening of the chest is very common, and is often associated with the stooping shoulders and arched back so commonly seen in rickety subjects.

Cranial signs.—These are only second

to the chest signs in frequency and importance. Of the eight hundred rickety children :

Both cranial and beaded ribs were present in 70 per cent.

Beaded ribs alone were present in 24 per cent.

Cranial signs alone were present in 6 per cent.

In the early months of infancy, when rickets is in active progress, the cranium typically has a somewhat expanded appearance as if the bones were thinned out. The widely open fontanelle and the thin skin with the blue veins showing through over the prominent forehead form a characteristic picture. When we have to deal with children of school age, the expanded appearance is lost, and the head is now massive-looking, and gives an impression as if the bones were greatly thickened, as is usually the case, especially along the lines of the sutures. There is a characteristic heaping up of bone in the region of the anterior fontanelle, and from that in a somewhat broad band along the line of the coronal suture. Often the whole frontal bone appears thickened, and the forehead prominent and projecting, but there is not the same tendency to bossing on the frontal region as in congenital syphilis. Very common and striking is the bossing over the parietal regions behind, which forms one of the most characteristic and persistent signs of rickets in the child's skull (Fig. 1).

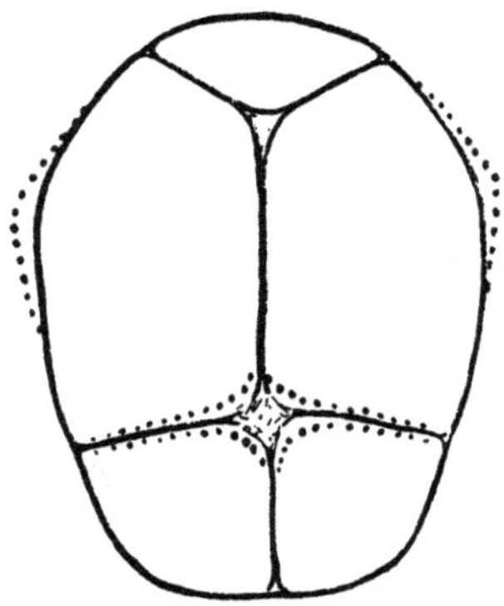

FIG. 1.—Infant skull showing position of parietal bossing and the thickening along the coronal suture, the characteristic cranial signs of rickets.

Tonsils and adenoids.—Tonsils and adenoids are commonly associated with rickets. Thus, of eight hundred rickety cases, 21 per cent. suffered from either enlarged tonsils or adenoids.

Of these children suffering from either tonsils or adenoids :

14	per cent.	had enlarged tonsils,
20	,,	had adenoids,
66	,,	had both conditions.

Anæmia was found to be marked in 20 per cent. of the rickety children.

Catarrh.—Associated with the conditions of tonsils and adenoids and anæmia is that of catarrh, which was carefully inquired into, to ascertain what influence rickets might have in producing catarrhal conditions likely to predispose to tubercle. Catarrh was present in 18 per cent. of the rickety children, mostly cases of persistent bronchial catarrh and nasal catarrh, the bronchial condition being much the more common. Cases of acute coryza and ordinary coughs and colds which might be accidental were not included. These catarrhal defects were common amongst Jewish children, but still more so amongst the poorer Christian children. This difference in favour of the Jewish children is possibly due to their good fat nutrition, which tends to prevent their developing catarrhal conditions.

Other defects associated with rickets.—Of other defects, several were characteristic, but were not present in sufficient numbers to be set down in percentage results. Stooping shoulders and lateral curvature are common, though, as already stated, the slighter forms of lateral curvature are more often suggested by flattening at one apex and prominence of the opposite side of the chest, with raising of one shoulder, than by an actual examination of the spine itself. Syphilis and rheumatism were exceptionally found in a few cases. Whilst pulmonary tubercle was not often found, enlargement of the submaxillary and cervical glands was common. This enlargement of the glands was usually of a discrete or shotty nature, and glandular abscesses of the neck were quite infrequent. This enlargement, indeed, is a part of the general hypertrophy which in rickets takes place in the whole of the lymphoid tissue, lymphatic system, and spleen. A very characteristic defect, present fairly frequently, was a harsh, dry condition of the skin, especially over the back of the upper arm and the back of the shoulders, but not infrequently extending over the whole body and face. As a rule this condition was associated with coarse, dry, lustreless hair, which was often scanty.

III

THE TEETH IN RICKETS

CHAPTER III

THE TEETH IN RICKETS

DEFECT in the calcium metabolism, especially in the laying down of calcium salts throughout the skeleton, is the most prominent feature in rickets, and the one responsible for most of the physical signs which mark the disease. Nowhere is this factor more marked than in the teeth. In rickets caries is exceedingly common, and hypoplasia, or defective calcification of the enamel, is well marked. A hypoplastic condition of the teeth[1] is characterized to the naked eye by a defective formation of the enamel and frequently stunted growth of the teeth. There may be only a pitting, producing a honeycombed

[1] "The Teeth in Rickets." *Proceedings of the Royal Society of Medicine*, 1916, vol. ix. (Section for the Study of Disease in Children), pp. 83–89.

appearance of the enamel, or the enamel covering is slight, and the cutting edge of the teeth presents sharp points, giving a characteristic appearance to the tooth. The defect usually extends from the cutting edge and may, in severe cases, involve the whole crown. As in syphilis, the condition is found typically in the permanent dentition, but whereas notched incisors and the contracted first molars of syphilis are but rarely met with in school children, the hypoplastic teeth of rickets are common. In everyday life one constantly sees these teeth and notes how well they often last. Thus frequently a smoker is seen whose teeth have been worn down in depth, and only short stumpy teeth are left, with a layer of enamel all round the cutting edge and the dentine exposed in the centre of the biting edge.

The calcification of the teeth begins about the fifth month of intra-uterine life, and the following diagrams (*see* p. 39) give the rate of progress of calcification at various periods for both the temporary and permanent teeth.

The only teeth of the permanent set which show any signs of calcification at birth are the cusps of the first molars. Fig. 3 shows the portion of the enamel which has undergone calcification at the end of the first two years of life, and the parts affected by the commonest form of hypoplasia. In the typical form of hypoplasia commonly met with, the teeth affected are the central and lateral incisors, the tips of the canines, and the crown of the first molars. The condition is symmetrical, affecting both jaws. Usually the depth of the defect is greater in the enamel of the central incisors than of the lateral incisors, and it will be noted that the enamel affected is identical with that laid during the first two years. This condition is pathognomonic of rickets. Rickets is the only condition which interferes with the deposition of calcium over this prolonged period.

In cases of acute illness, especially fevers, the finger-nails are apt to show grooves marking the state of depressed growth of the cells of the bed of the nail during the progress of the disease. In the case of the teeth, a groove more or less broad, or even a succession of grooves with healthy enamel in between, may mark attacks of grave illness in the child. Frequently without a history, a shrewd guess can be made at the period of occurrence of some serious illness by the part of the enamel of the teeth which is affected. But it is usually a grave and prolonged illness which thus leaves its mark, more especially measles, followed by whooping-cough. Scarlet fever is less likely to have this effect.

Hypoplasia due to congenital syphilis is rare, whilst the form due to rickets is exceedingly common among school children. At birth calcification has involved the crowns of the deciduous incisors, the cusps of the deciduous canines and deciduous molars, and the tips of the cusps of the first permanent molars. The portions of the temporary enamel not yet calcified at birth in the temporary set frequently suffer from hypoplasia. Any disturbance in the function of the ameloblasts, the cells which, according to Tomes, either secrete the

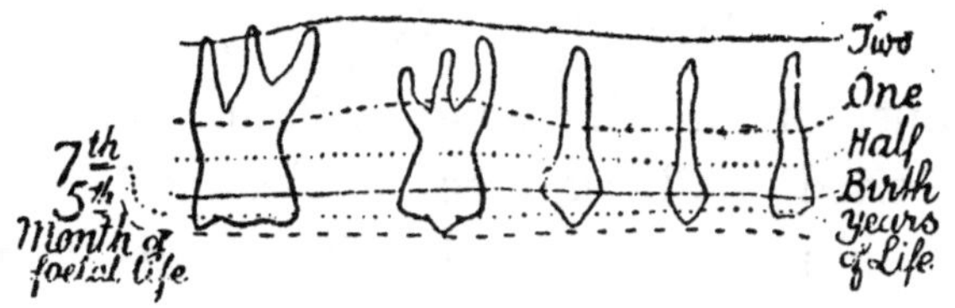

FIG. 1.—Showing calcification of temporary teeth at various periods.

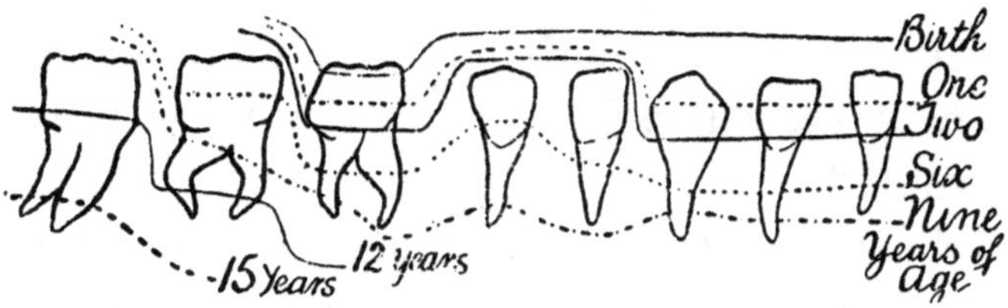

FIG. 2.—Showing calcification of permanent teeth at various periods.

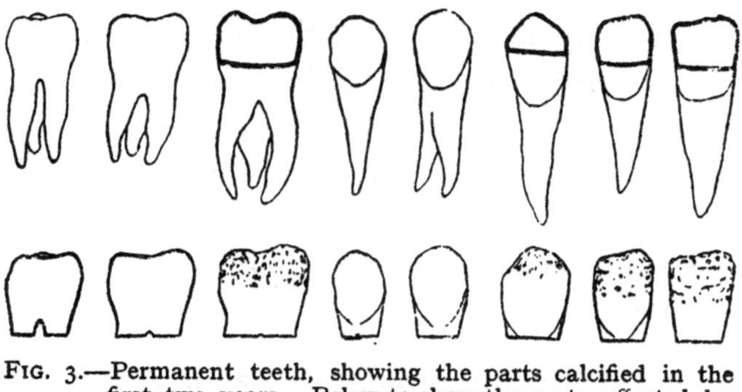

FIG. 3.—Permanent teeth, showing the parts calcified in the first two years Below to show the parts affected by commonest form of hypoplasia.

enamel or in which the calcium salts are deposited, will lead to the enamel being thin in parts and to the lime salts being imperfectly laid down, so that the compact enamel is more easily disintegrated. In other words, the agents which determine the tendency to decay are those which affect the soft enamel organ in the earliest history of the tooth and not those which affect the enamel after the tooth has been erupted.

Seafaring communities are said to have good teeth, and this is generally attributed to the action of ozone and pure air. But more likely causes are the favourable conditions under which the children of such communities are brought up in early life, as regards fresh air, sunlight and ventilation. Professor Keith, in his fascinating book on *The Antiquity of Man* (p. 12), speaking of the Coldrum collection of Neolithic men, draws a comparison between Neolithic and modern man as regards their teeth :—

Amongst modern Kentish folk, as is the case all over modern Britain, there is a tendency to crowding and irregularities of the teeth ; the palate and jaws do not grow and expand sufficiently in youth to give room for a symmetrical eruption of the teeth. . . . The nose is narrow and the palate contracted, and its vault is high. The teeth are not worn down as in Neolithic men ; they are very liable to be attacked by caries. The front teeth, when the jaws are closed, do not meet edge to edge as in primitive races ; like the blades of scissors, they overlap, the lower passing behind the upper. In the Neolithic people all these modern characters are absent. Abscesses or gumboils at the roots of the deeply ground teeth were, however, common ; but there is not a single carious tooth to be seen in the Coldrum collection. The teeth are regular in their arrangement, the palates were well formed, but in actual size the teeth possess the same dimensions as those of modern English people. All these changes, which are appearing in the teeth and jaws of modern British people, arise, we suppose, from the soft nature of our modern diet. We believe that were modern men to resume a Neolithic diet their teeth and palates would again be moulded in the ancient manner.

The difference is, however, hardly capable of such easy solution. Rickets was probably a disease unknown among Neolithic infants, as is largely the case among savage races to-day, notwithstanding frequent privations as regards food. Contrast the life of Neolithic men living under primitive conditions, rising with the sun and going to rest at sunset, and living in small communities scattered over wide areas, with that of the slum conditions under which so large a proportion of our population lives to-day. It is not a question of food, but of the deprivation of fresh air, exercise and sunlight, which profoundly alters the metabolism of the child and produces aberration in the growth not only of the bones and teeth, but in probably every tissue of the body. Natural selection is not always beneficial in its action. Nature is ever mindful of the continuity of the race, and if the slum-dweller is essential for its continuity an individual capable of adapting himself to such conditions will undoubtedly be produced.

In judging of the presence of hypoplasia, it was found practically impossible to make accurate observations on the temporary teeth of infants of school age. Caries was so universal and extensive that it completely masked the hypoplasia. It was evident that a hypoplastic condition of the teeth was common in the temporary set, and was, in all probability, the chief factor in bringing about premature decay. For the purposes of statistics only the records of the permanent dentition have been taken, and in marking a case as one of hypoplasia, only the severer forms are admitted, and cases of slight pitting, chalky-looking patches in the enamel, and so on have been excluded, although microscopically such teeth would be found markedly defective and liable to disintegration. Of the 586 rickety cases in which a record of the permanent teeth could be taken, 42 per cent. had normal teeth and 58 per cent. had defective teeth; 20 per cent. of these showed hypoplasia frequently combined with decay, and 38 per cent. had decayed teeth. This is not equivalent to saying that 42 per cent. of school children have normal teeth. As already pointed out, all infants with a record only of temporary teeth have been excluded, because these teeth were so universally decayed as to make accurate observations on the structure impossible. Again, most of the children with records of the permanent teeth were about the ages of twelve or thirteen years, when all the permanent teeth have been erupted except the third molars, and caries has had least time to make its appearance. It is a somewhat quaint commentary on the general state of the teeth of the community to be compelled to explain why only 58 per cent. are given as having defective teeth.

Of the cases with carious teeth, the lower first molar was decayed in 80 per cent., the upper first molar was decayed in 30 per cent., one or more lower premolars in 30 per cent., and one or more upper premolars in 12·5 per cent. The incisors, canines, and second molars were seldom decayed. The shape of the incisors and canines must protect them from many of the causes of decay to which the flattened grinding molars are subjected. The lower first molars decay out of all proportion to the others, and their earlier eruption is not a sufficient explanation of this. It is to be attributed rather to the main part of the enamel of the crown having been laid down in the first two years of life, when rickety conditions are operative. Naturally the lower teeth, which lie in the well of the mouth, will suffer more seriously from deleterious influences which surround the teeth.

Even though no macroscopic change indicative of hypoplasia is to be found in these teeth, in all probability their microscopic character is distinctly affected. One practical point may be noted. Frequently, on looking into a child's mouth, the two milk molars or the first permanent molar will be seen with blackened exposed dentine and the enamel on the surface of the crown removed. Closer examination will show that these are still effective teeth and that there is no pyorrhœa or gum irritation around them. The surface of the tooth can be freely touched with the spatula. The dentine of the tooth seems to have become consolidated, and usually, though the teeth do not look well, they can be safely left, the process of decay having become arrested. Frequently it is not a process of decay in the ordinary sense, for the thin defective enamel on the surface of the crowns of the grinding teeth can sometimes be seen breaking off in distinct flakes. Many of the conditions conducive to rickets are present in the parents of these children, and *a priori* it might be expected that this would frequently be a congenital defect. In such a case in a certain proportion of children the milk incisors should show hypoplastic changes. The enamel of the crown of the milk incisors begins to be laid down about the seventeenth week, half-way through intra-uterine life, and has progressed to a considerable extent at the time of birth. At birth, half the crowns of the incisors, the tips of the canines and the cusps of the molars are calcified in the temporary set, and by about six months after birth the calcification of the crowns is completed. Careful search for a hypoplastic condition of the milk incisors during a long period both in school children and in the babies who have attended Infant Welfare Centres has failed to detect a case. It is strong presumptive evidence that rickets is not a congenital condition, and is another instance of the care that

Nature takes that, whatever else suffers, the germ at least is protected during intra-uterine life.

A later form of hypoplasia is every now and then seen in which the two premolars and the second molars are affected, whilst the incisors, canines, and first molars are not affected. This later form of hypoplasia must be due to influences acting on the child from the second to the sixth year. Association has been recognized between lamellar cataract and hypoplastic teeth. Mr. Norman Bennett collected twenty-two cases of lamellar cataract, all of which showed well-defined hypoplasia in the permanent teeth, and in thirteen cases there was a history of convulsions whilst teething.

An interesting observation is made by Fleischman that the teeth of all the persons he examined who had a history of infantile tetany showed hypoplasia of the enamel.

IV

SOME FURTHER OBSERVATIONS ON THE TEETH

D

CHAPTER IV

SOME FURTHER OBSERVATIONS ON THE TEETH

IF one hundred better-class children living under good social conditions are compared with one hundred poorly fed children living under slum conditions, even a casual inspection will show that the teeth of the poorly fed and badly housed children are much more defective than those of the better fed ones.

Another inquiry was made as to the teeth conditions in 403 children taken from the ordinary London County Council schools.[1] All these children were eleven years and over, and of the 403 children, 281 were taken from schools where the general conditions as regards feeding and housing were

[1] "Abnormal Conditions of the Enamel in Cases of Malnutrition." *Lancet*, Oct. 5, 1918, p. 456.

distinctly below the average, whilst in 122 these conditions were relatively good. No attempt was made to select children of poor nutrition beyond that they belonged to a poor school and lived under slum conditions in poor and overcrowded neighbourhoods, such as Bethnal Green and Shoreditch. As a contrast 122 children were taken from good-class schools in North London, where the social conditions were fairly good, and where the general state of nutrition was good. The following results were obtained :—

(A) 403 children. (B) 281 where nutrition was decidedly poor. (C) 122 children of good nutrition.

	(A) Cases.	(A) Per cent.	(B) Cases.	(B) Per cent.	(C) Cases.	(C) Per cent.
Enamel normal ..	273	=67·5	167	=60	106	=87
,, defective	130	=32·5	114	=40	16	=13

Carious conditions have not been dealt with in these figures. The conditions of the enamel met with in these cases may be summarized as follows :—

1. *Typical hypoplasia.*—This has already been dealt with in the last chapter.

2. *Honeycombed teeth.*—This condition is much the same as the first, except that the deficiency in the enamel leads to the formation of small depressed pits scattered over the surface of the teeth, giving a very characteristic appearance.

3. *Horizontal bands of thickened enamel and transverse grooves in the enamel,* indicating acute illnesses of a more or less prolonged nature. Short acute illnesses seem less likely to produce this condition than prolonged debilitating conditions, such as measles, especially when followed by whooping-cough.

4. *Chalky appearance of the enamel,* varying from white patches or transverse bands on the surface of the enamel to a general opacity affecting its whole surface. This is a very well-marked defect, and the contrast which this condition gives with the clear semi-transparency of healthy enamel is one of the chief things that strike the observer in the teeth of poorly nourished children. As will be seen, it is the commonest defect found in malnutrition.

5. *Brown lines of Retzius* or brown

staining of the enamel is a common and well-marked defect found in cases of malnutrition. This defect may be found as a brown line running as a rule across the incisors, and, it may be, the canines. It may be a brown patch of varying size and intensity of colouring, though it is usually a rusty brown. Very commonly it is associated with marked opacity of the enamel, and it seems to indicate a somewhat severe degree of disturbance of the nutrition.

Placing the frequency of occurrence in the poor-class and the better-class children side by side, the following is the result given in percentages :—

	In 281 poor-class children.	In 122 good-class children.
	Per cent.	Per cent.
Opaque chalky enamel ..	28·5	9
Brown line of Retzius ..	13·0	1 case
Hypoplasia	8·5	5
Honeycombed teeth ..	2·5	0

As already shown, out of 281 poor children, 114, or 40 per cent., had defective enamel, as compared with 13 per cent.

amongst the better-class children. Taking the 114 cases with defective enamel among the poorer-class children there was found:

	Per cent.
Chalky enamel	80=70
Brown lines of Retzius	38=33
Typical hypoplasia	24=21
Honeycombed teeth	7= 6

It is of great importance to note the teeth most commonly affected. In the children where the enamel was opaque and chalky the teeth were affected in the following order of frequency:—

	Per cent.		Per cent.
Central incisors ..	78	Premolars ..	20
Lateral incisors ..	55	First molars ..	10
Canines	30	Second molars ..	5

These figures are accurate except in the case of the first and second molars. The first molars were frequently badly decayed or the tooth had been extracted. The second molars in many of these cases had not yet been erupted.

In thirty-eight cases when the teeth showed the brown lines of Retzius:

	Per cent.
Central incisors affected in	36=95
Lateral " " "	11=29
Canines affected in	5=13
First molar	1 case

It is important to note that in hypoplasia and in cases where the chalky patches and the brown lines of Retzius were found the teeth which suffered chiefly were, first, the central incisors; secondly, the lateral incisors; and, thirdly, the canines in this order of frequency. Reference to the diagram will show that the calcification of the enamel of the crowns of these teeth goes on during the first two years of the child's life. So that these defects are due to errors of nutrition affecting the child at this early period when the rate of growth, and notably that of the brain, is relatively enormous.

V

THE MENTAL DEVELOPMENT IN RICKETS

THE ENDOCRINOUS GLANDS AND RICKETS

CHAPTER V

THE MENTAL DEVELOPMENT IN RICKETS. THE ENDOCRINOUS GLANDS AND RICKETS

THERE is a general impression that the rickety child is precocious, but in reality it is essentially a backward child. In considering the development of these one thousand children, it was found that of the eight hundred who showed signs of rickets :

	Per cent.
Walking or speech was delayed in ..	48·0
Both being delayed in	29·0
Walking alone delayed in	12·5
Speech alone delayed in	6·5
Neither speech nor walking delayed in	52·0

The period constituting delay is taken as eighteen months, so that those cases of delayed development did not walk or speak till after the age of eighteen months.

The mental state of the rickety child may be considered: (1) During the active stage of the disease, from six months to two years; (2) at the time of entry into school; (3) in later school life.

During the acute stage from six months to two years.—Normally the healthy child rejoices in activity. The mental condition of the rickety child is essentially a placid one. The infant suffering from active rickets is too much engaged with the struggle for life to have time to fret about lesser things. It does not expend its energy in crying, for it is wholly occupied in getting sufficient oxygen into its lungs to supply its present needs. The mechanical act of respiration is a laboured effort which exhausts the child's energies. The only time it is apt to be fretful is when it is moved; when left alone it is placid and silent. But though the physical condition of the child demands that it should conserve its energies, the nervous system is by no means placid. Laryngismus stridulus and convulsions are common. Out of 50 cases of laryngismus, Dr. Gee found that 48 were rickety, and of these 19 had general convulsions. Out of 102 children in whom general convulsions occurred, 46 were rickety—that is about half. Incontinence is a symptom that is of frequent occurrence in rickets, and it is of interest to note that thyroid treatment is frequently successful in these cases. The mental progress of the child is slow, and this is especially shown in speech, as already noted. Defective forms of speech are frequent; lalling is common, and stammering and stuttering are apt to develop later. The child has difficulty in picking up new words.

Mental state at time of entry into school.—At school age the rickety child is distinctly backward when compared with the normal child. The backwardness may last for some years, and then somewhat suddenly the child often makes a rapid advance noticeable to both parents and teachers. There is, as it were, a sudden intellectual awakening. This is characteristic of the mentality of rickets. Typically the child at school age is dull, and its powers of attention are poor, rendering it the despair of its teacher. By the fourth or fifth year of life the child is beginning to improve physically and to become more active; but the mental improvement does not begin till somewhat later. The mother frequently makes the statement that all her children begin to pick up wonderfully about the age of seven, an observation which is quite consistent with the facts in the great majority of cases. Why this should be will be seen later.

Mental condition in later school life.—In the slighter forms of rickets, and especially when the natural conditions become more favourable, the child's mental condition may return to the normal, and no permanent damage seems to be done. But in a large number of cases the sudden progress which the child makes only carries it to a certain limit still below the normal, so that its capacity is only equal to that of a child two or three years younger. The child's powers of attention and concentration remain poor, the mental response is much delayed, and frequently a question will have to be repeated several times before the child grasps what has been said. In the ordinary work of the class the child remains a distinct drag. A judicious selection of such children and the placing of them together in a class where they can be put to modelling in the round, drawing with coloured chalks, and, in the case of girls, housework, is often followed with the happiest results. For the first time the child does work which it can really do well; a few weeks at such work, where the hand assists the brain, will often convert a dull, listless child into one that is bright and alert. Its self-respect is increased as it finds that at certain kinds of work it can hold its own. The training of the mind through the muscular sense is peculiarly well adapted to this type of child. When the mental condition remains below the normal, the child in severer cases is apt to be moody, and is not infrequently vicious and spiteful, and uncertain in temper. Such cases are especially troublesome, as they are often associated with children of younger age than themselves owing to their slow progress through the standards. In many cases the early struggle against adverse circumstances leads to a certain infirmity of purpose which persists through adult life, and probably accounts for a good many half failures in adult life.

Dividing the eight hundred rickety children into three classes—bright, average, and backward, it was found that :

11 per cent. could be considered bright.
64 ,, ,, ,, average.
25 ,, ,, ,, backward.

The very universality of the condition probably makes one content with not only a much lower general standard of mental development, but also with a lower standard of growth than might legitimately be expected if the environment of the child were such as to allow of its full mental and physical development. Speaking of standard measurements for school children, Dr. Kerr very rightly remarks[1]: " As a nation we should not accept quietly the difference in physique between primary and

[1] "Standard Measurements for School Children," by James Kerr, M.A., M.D. *School Hygiene*, April 1918.

secondary schools. We must make all our children pass into the one national standard of physique, and no longer regard as inevitable the inferior physique of artisans, and superior of professional classes, knowing that the difference is largely due to social failure and an index of national inefficiency." There is then recognizable a certain type of child, which may be fat and well nourished, though the muscular tone and development are defective, often markedly so. The conditions associated with the rickety child are strongly suggestive of hypothyroidism.[1] These may be detailed as follows :—

1. Coarseness of features and pale pasty complexion.
2. Tendency to adenoids and catarrhal conditions associated with general lymphatic enlargement.
3. Nocturnal incontinence peculiarly amenable to treatment by thyroid extract.
4. Tendency to laryngismus stridulus

[1] "On Some Signs and Symptoms of Hypothyroidism in School Children." *Lancet*, Sept, 5, 1914.

and general convulsions so often associated with defective calcium metabolism.

5. Pronounced harshness of the skin.
6. Coarse scanty hair, without lustre.
7. Backwardness of speech and slow general mental development.
8. Softness and enlargement of the bones at the epiphyseal ends and thickening of the membranous bone of the shaft of the long bones and of the flat bones of the skull.
9. Hypoplasia and other defects of the enamel, with marked tendency to caries.

In the present state of our knowledge of the action of the endocrinous glands it is impossible to be dogmatic in our statements as to the part they play in growth and development. From early infancy the thyroid apparatus, including the parathyroids under this term, and the thymus seem to have an important influence in regulating the growth and development of the tissues, and the action of these two systems seems closely correlated. It is noteworthy that these glands have a common origin, the thyroid being developed as an outgrowth from the fore gut or buccal epithelium ventrally to the branchial arches, whilst the parathyroid and thymus are developed from the epithelium of the third and fourth branchial arches themselves. The signs and symptoms just enumerated suggest diminished action of the thyroid apparatus associated with increased action of the thymus. It seems as if the restraining action of the thyroid being lessened the influence of the thymus tends to predominate. It can be readily understood that the gland most likely to be affected adversely by bad housing conditions would be the thyroid, which is so dependent on a free arterial circulation and rapid oxidation to meet the many demands made on its economy. Possibly the strain placed upon the thyroid gland by such infections as measles and whooping-cough may so exhaust the glands as to lead to diminished thyroid and parathyroid action and consequent disturbance in calcium metabolism, leading to certain forms of hypoplasia already described as liable to occur in these diseases.

Later in life the gonads and the pituitary gland seem to play a large part in the growth of the tissues, the thyroid continuing an important controlling factor, whilst the action of the thymus rapidly diminishes. Of the interrelationship of the various glands little is known, but there is reason to believe that the thyroid remains a dominant factor throughout life, and that any agent which interferes with its activities tends to throw out of action the great controlling gland of the whole endocrinous system. In the growing child rickets may be considered as a phase of hypothyroidism induced by the bad hygienic conditions under which the great mass of the slum population is brought up.

VI

THE CAUSATION OF RICKETS

CHAPTER VI

THE CAUSATION OF RICKETS

THE controversy as to the conditions which produce rickets still remains unsettled, and in this period of reconstruction it assumes a very vital importance. For if defective or deficient feeding alone is responsible for the production of rickets, then the solution of the problem, as already stated, should be comparatively simple. Much stress has lately been laid on the accessory food factors, the vitamines, in the causation of disease. This deficiency disease can be best studied in tropical countries, notably in the case of polished rice as the cause of beri-beri, where the absence of certain accessory food factors is the essential etiological agent. It can be readily understood that when a diet consists very largely of one article, such as rice, the complete removal of the vitamines which pertains to the polishing of the rice may be productive of the most dire results. Our knowledge of these accessory food factors is but small, but two facts seem probable: firstly, that the actual amount of these vitamines necessary to keep the body in health is very small, and secondly, that these accessory factors are very widespread in the various articles of food which form our ordinary dietary. Even in the most defective forms of feeding in this country it is doubtful if deficiency in the vitamines is likely to be a serious factor affecting the nutrition of the child. In his experiments on lion cubs at the Zoological Gardens, Sir John Bland Sutton drew attention to the importance of cod-liver oil in the prevention of rickets. Lately Dr. and Mrs. Mellanby, in some valuable experiments on the feeding of dogs, have laid great stress on the absence of the vitamine Fat Soluble A, contained in cod-liver oil, butter, and to a less extent in other fats, as an important factor, possibly the essential factor, in the production of rickets. These observations have received the support of Professor Hopkins, who states the case still more strongly when he says[1]: "I am convinced rickets arises when fat soluble vitamine is deficient in the food. Other factors, such as a general deficient hygiene, may be contributory, but I, for one, am convinced that the dietetic error is the primary cause." There is a danger in dissociating laboratory work from clinical observation, and there is always a difficulty in reproducing in the laboratory the conditions which pertain to natural conditions. Such observations have to be received with caution. The environment of lion cubs born in captivity in England is so inimical to the growth of the organism that the mere fact that the administration of cod-liver oil enabled a few of these animals to be successfully reared cannot be taken as evidence that cod-liver oil prevents rickets. In Dr. and Mrs. Mellanby's experiments it must be remembered

[1] "The Practical Importance of Vitamines," by Professor F. Gowland Hopkins. *British Medical Journal*, April 26, 1919, p. 507.

that the growth and development of the dog are very rapid, and the effects of the dietary were rapidly produced in the space of five or six weeks, when the animals were killed. The effects of the severe dietary was evidently disastrous to a degree to the whole nutrition of the animal. So much was this the case, that these observers found great difficulty in preventing these animals succumbing to intercurrent disease. It is claimed with truth that, in these experiments, severe conditions of hypoplasia were produced in dogs, whilst on a fat-free diet in the space of a few weeks. There is no doubt of the hypoplasia produced; indeed, it is of a type so severe that its like is not met with in the human subject. Most of the defective conditions of the enamel detailed in previous chapters were associated with rickets, but, as was pointed out, a certain proportion, notably the band or ring defects in the enamel, were due to intercurrent disease, notably measles associated with whooping-cough. In children it may be said that any disturbance of the growth and nutrition of the child which is severe and long continued may, if it acts during the period when the calcium is being actively laid down by the ameloblasts, result in defect in that process leading to hypoplasia. In the typical form of hypoplasia which affects the central and lateral incisors, the tips of the canines and the crowns of the first molars, rickets is the one condition which interferes with the deposition of calcium over this prolonged period, namely, the first two years of the child's life, and the presence of this defect is pathognomonic of the disease. In the experiments of Dr. and Mrs. Mellanby the dogs undoubtedly suffered from a disease in which the long bones showed extreme rickety changes and from severe hypoplasia of a type never seen in the child, but it would be dangerous to infer from this that the dietary, which was apparently responsible for these conditions, is the usual factor in producing rickets as met with in children. Other observers on the same lines have come to a different conclusion. Leonard Findlay found in an experimental investigation on the etiology of rickets in young dogs[1] that puppies freely exercised, when fed on bread and water and oatmeal and water, did not develop rickets but became marasmic and died, and, later, Dr. Noel Paton, in association with Dr. Findlay and Dr. Watson, in a further experimental inquiry[2] into the same subject, came to the following conclusion: "Pups kept in the country and freely exercised in the open air, although they had actually a smaller amount of milk fat than those kept in the laboratory, remained free of rickets, while the animals kept in the laboratory all became rickety." There are many arguments against the theory that deficiency of the vitamines is the essential cause of rickets. The observations already detailed in the second chapter indicate very strongly that the absence of Fat Soluble A is not the prime cause. Out of one thousand children 81·4 per cent. were breast fed, and of the remaining

[1] "The Etiology of Rickets," by Leonard Findlay. *British Medical Journal*, July 4, 1908, p. 13.

[2] "Observations on the Cause of Rickets," by D. Noel Paton, Leonard Findlay, and Alex. Watson. *British Medical Journal*, Dec. 7, 1918, p. 625.

18·6 per cent. practically all were brought up on cow's milk. This was carefully elicited from the mothers. An important factor in the enquiry was that the mothers were asked to attend with the child at the time of the examination, and about three-fourths of the mothers actually did attend. The enquiry was made just prior to the war, and the general nutrition of these Jewish mothers was good and their fat nutrition was excellent. Yet notwithstanding these facts, that 81·4 per cent. of these healthy mothers, living on wholesome food with an ample variety, suckled their children, whilst 18·6 per cent. were brought up on cow's milk, eight hundred out of the one thousand children showed the stigmata of rickets. So forcibly has the state of good nutrition of many of these rickety children thrust itself on the attention of some observers, that they actually consider rickets to be due to overfeeding. As already stated, rickets is a disease which notably tends towards recovery. This does not apply only to Jewish children but to the non-Jewish as well, where actual deficient feeding is usually associated with defective housing conditions. Why should a child improve, as these children usually do, at from three to seven years of age? There is no improvement in the dietary. Less milk is given to the child than in infancy, and a real difficulty in feeding is created by the fact that the child shows a positive dislike to milk and will avoid taking it whenever possible. The improvement is probably due to the fact that the child's environment at this time becomes more natural. The mother of these poor families has but little time to take the child out during the first two to three years of its existence, and the child cannot go out without the mother. It is a statement commonly made by mothers that all their children are delicate up to the age of five or seven, and that they then seem definitely to improve in health and become stronger. There is probably a large foundation of truth in this, for at this age the child becomes to a large extent independent of parental authority and is allowed to lead a relatively more healthy and natural existence by being given the freedom of the streets and of the open air. But by this time, unfortunately, much irreparable damage has been done. Our climate is a trying one, and during the short days of our long winter many hours out of the twenty-four must necessarily be spent indoors in the case of children. With such a climate it is all the more essential that ample space and proper ventilation, with provision for the maintenance of bodily warmth, should be provided in our houses.

It is interesting to note that in Italy, South Africa, and Australia, where there is abundance of sunshine and life is much in the open, rickets does not develop, though the conditions as regards feeding are often very defective. There is no race immunity. Italians in the slums of London and of New York suffer severely from rickets, though both the quality and the quantity of the food are much better than they would be in their own country. Australia is beginning of late years to develop rickets in proportion as the towns grow in size and density of population.

Again, rickets is by no means confined to the slum-dweller. As already noted, a mild form of rickets is fairly common amongst the children of wealthy parents, where the feeding of the child is beyond reproach and malt and cod-liver oil form one of the staple articles of diet. These children are thought to be delicate, and they are accordingly pampered in closed rooms and deprived of proper air and exercise. The weight of evidence shows that defective housing and over-crowding and the slum conditions under which the children live, with the loss of fresh air, sunshine, and exercise which these conditions entail, are the essential factors in producing rickets. The great majority of the children from whom these statistics were taken lived in two- or three-roomed houses, frequently in one room, and in one of these rooms the cooking and ordinary household work was carried on. Such conditions will inevitably produce rickets whether the food be good or bad.

VII

THE REMEDY

F

CHAPTER VII

THE REMEDY

WHATEVER the part played by the vitamines in the production of disease in England, it is evidently of the first importance that the part they play in the economy of the system should be carefully studied. But it is of more than academic interest to try to come to an early solution of the problem as to whether defective housing or deficient feeding is the essential factor in retarding the growth and proper development of the nation. If the condition were due almost entirely to deficiency of vitamines, the solution of the problem would be easy, for rationing the nation is a process of which we have now considerable experience, and that at a time when foodstuffs were scarce and substitutes of all kinds were common.

When the world's food market is again well stored the process would be easy and effective, and if this were all that were required it would be well to concentrate on this and not to spend many millions on housing schemes which could wait for a more leisurely treatment. It is difficult to avoid the conclusion, the converse of that arrived at by Professor Hopkins, that defective housing and slum dwellings are the essential causes of rickets, whilst deficient feeding is a contributory and aggravating factor, and that any scheme of feeding, however perfect, will inevitably be a failure so long as slums and housing conditions are left as they are. In emphasizing the importance of proper housing the defect in feeding must not be lost sight of. It is a matter worthy of note that it is of little use giving malt and cod-liver oil to children who are suffering from lack of food. For some years now malt and cod-liver oil have been supplied fairly freely in many of the London County Council schools to poorly fed children, and with but very indifferent results. What is of much greater help to these children is a fair supply of milk, and if this could be given twice daily, half a pint in the middle of the morning and another half-pint in the middle of the afternoon, the greatest benefit would result. The difficulty is that the administration of malt and cod-liver oil is comparatively easy, whilst the giving of milk takes time and involves labour. The head mistress has not time for this, but if capable women were placed in control of the milk supply it could be carried out on a large scale with the greatest benefit to these badly nourished children. The right of the young infant as regards milk supply should also be guarded. At the infant welfare clinics, when a quart of milk is necessary for the child, the mother frequently tells the physician that it is impossible to obtain this quantity, and that, though she does her best, she cannot afford to get more than half or one pint. The mother will tell this quite frankly and without bitterness, as if it were part of the scheme of existence that such hard cases as hers should occur. Such a state of affairs is discreditable, and should no longer be tolerated. Even if the fault lies with the parent, and usually it does not, the State should see to it that each child has an adequate supply of whatever foodstuffs the physician, who is examining the child on the State's behalf, deems necessary.

The negligence of some parents may demand correction or punishment, but care must be taken that the child does not suffer in the meantime through the parents' want of care. The supervision of the child must begin with the expectant mother, and should be continued systematically by one competent authority throughout infancy and school age till the child has reached its full development. Such a scheme is already well in hand and should not be difficult to carry out. But no scheme which rests content with this will do much to advance the public health unless large measures are taken to deal with the question of housing. The facts as regards defective housing are not now in dispute. Such facts as those brought out by Dr. Maxwell Williamson, where the incidence of pulmonary tuberculosis in relation to size of houses in Edinburgh in 1912 is shown as follows, speak for themselves.[1]

RATE OF INCIDENCE.

	Per 1,000 inhabitants.
1 Room	6·9
2 Rooms	5·6
3 Rooms	3·5
4 Rooms and over	1·4

It is self-evident that the remedy is not to build sanatoria, but to demolish slums. The census of 1911 shows that 7,000,000 persons, nearly one-sixth of the total population of the kingdom, lived in one-, two-, or three-roomed houses. The problem is a tremendous one, but our ideas as regards what can be done in the way of raising money have changed of late, and the question of the abolition of slum tenements and the substitution of proper housing throughout the country must be treated on broad legislative lines. Individual enterprise cannot cope with it. The question of transport enters largely into

[1] "Housing and Tuberculosos." *The British Journal of Tuberculosis*, July 1915.

the subject, and forms a sound argument for the nationalization of all the means of transport. Whatever views are held as to the nationalization of the land, it can hardly be denied that each parent has a right to adequate space for the erection of a decent dwelling where he and his family can live in health and comfort. There is no justice in keeping such areas as Hampstead and Highgate as reserves for the rich, whilst the poor have to crowd, as best they can, into slum dwellings at an exorbitant rental in such areas as Hoxton, Shoreditch, Bethnal Green, and Whitechapel. Garden City schemes, such as the late Canon Barnett's at Golder's Green, show what can be done in the way of mingling houses of low rental with houses for the wealthy without destroying the amenities of either.

Belgium before the war had gone a long way towards settling the problem by the erection of cheap working-class houses in the country, with little plots of ground for cultivation, and by introducing a cheap and rapid service of trains for carrying the workman to and from work. At one sweep the Peabody Fund in London has profoundly altered the health conditions of the people, so that of the 22,000 persons housed under this scheme, with weekly average earnings for the head of the family of only 22s. 3d., the death-rate is only 10·4 as compared with 14·3 for the whole City of London. The London County Council has also carried out housing schemes which have shown excellent results. Not that such schemes are altogether healthy in their action, and may even be anti-social, in so far as they tend to crowd the population into the centres of the towns. These schemes, indeed, involve the writing off by the public body of the difference between the commercial value and the value for working-class dwellings of the site, so that the houses are offered at terms which involve the payment of a heavy subsidy from the ratepayers to their tenants. No such subsidy is offered for housing in outlying districts, which is the true solution.

There is a natural tendency in London for factories to take the place of slum dwellings. In one or two cases it has happened that the London County Council has actually built schools in crowded areas where this has taken place, and has had difficulty subsequently in filling these schools. This displacement of slum houses by factories has been quite noticeable of late years in such areas as Shoreditch, Stepney, Islington, and elsewhere, and is a process which might well be encouraged by lowering the heavy rates which often drive manufacturers to look further afield for sites where these are not so oppressive. Powers to acquire building sites at reasonable rates, active legislation limiting the number of houses to the acre, making it incumbent upon municipalities to see that every house is reasonably fit for habitation, requiring town planning and the extension of cheap travelling facilities to effect a proper distribution of the population, are problems lying to our hand which demand a speedy solution. Needless to say, no housing scheme will immediately rid our towns of slum areas. Indolence, intemperance, and thriftlessness are faults not to be at once eradicated by any housing scheme, however effective.

At the same time, the slums of to-day are by no means the slums of fifty or twenty-five years ago. There has been a steady improvement in the habits of the people, and the standard of living is on a higher and better scale. After the wonderful response our soldiers and the women of the empire have made to the nation's call in her time of need, it would be ungenerous to deny to any class of the community the opportunity to work out its own salvation in the direction of healthy living. Educating the child to proper ideas of how to live is very essential, and whilst there is much to be said against a conscript army, there is little to be said against conscripting the children and youth of the nation for health purposes. The Boy Scout movement might very well be adapted to a great national scheme whereby the young could be taught right and clean methods of living with a certain time spent annually in camp under discipline. At no time can discipline be so well or so profitably applied as it can to the young growing mind with its hopeful outlook and wide enthusiasms.

Drunkenness is by no means the venial offence it was fifty years ago, and no man can now be a decent member of society and offend against its ordinary conventions as regards sobriety. This is the growth of a few years. Similarly the pressure brought to bear on the slum-dweller by the presence of healthy and clean dwellings round him might well be expected to have a considerable influence in a few years in raising the standard of living throughout the whole community. At present we can say nothing, for it is idle to expect the slum-dweller to be thrifty and to save one or two shillings a week when his whole life is spent in continuous discomfort and misery, and the expenditure of these few shillings will obtain an immediate amelioration of his condition in the relative comfort and sociability of the public-house.

INDEX

For Product Safety Concerns and Information please contact our EU representative GPSR@taylorandfrancis.com
Taylor & Francis Verlag GmbH, Kaufingerstraße 24, 80331 München, Germany

www.ingramcontent.com/pod-product-compliance
Lightning Source LLC
LaVergne TN
LVHW021113300926
849160LV00009B/726

9781138100862